Adaptogens and Health Care

by

Anatoly G. Antoshechkin, M.D., Ph.D.

authorHOUSE™

1663 LIBERTY DRIVE, SUITE 200
BLOOMINGTON, INDIANA 47403
(800) 839-8640
WWW.AUTHORHOUSE.COM

First published by AuthorHouse 02/17/05

ISBN: 1-4208-2732-4 (e)
ISBN: 1-4208-2733-2 (sc)

Printed in the United States of America
Bloomington, Indiana

This book is printed on acid-free paper.

Table of Contents

INTRODUCTION

Despite advances in modern pharmacology—a science directed towards the curing of diseases by man-made drugs—it is obvious that the **prevention** of diseases (prophylaxis) is more reasonable approach to health care than the **treatment** of them. However creation of prophylactic remedy against any common disease has been appeared difficult. At the present time only vaccines are specific remedies prevented some infectious diseases. All others noninfectious common illnesses can't be effectively prevented by any pharmaceutical drug specified for particular disease.

Another approach to prophylaxis of sicknesses is to search for remedies that possess the capability to activate biochemical mechanisms, which are responsible for general human body resistance against some functional disturbances and development of common illnesses. The purpose of this book is to familiarize the reader with the basic knowledge about adaptogenic plants, some constituents of which restore the compromised activity of important physiological functions of the human organism and reduce the risk of development of many diseases.

Part I: The Initial Reason for Many Diseases

CHAPTER ONE
What is Stress?

In everyday language, the term stress usually means a human reaction to some sort of unpleasant situation or danger. The scientific sense of the term is much more complex. It is important to be more familiar with this sense because stress deteriorates whole number of processes in the body and is the initial reason for many diseases.

The stress concept was first introduced by Hans Selye in 1936. Since then, abundant experimental and clinical data has been brought forth that substantiate the theory of stress and define its underlying biochemical mechanisms.

Anatoly G. Antoshechkin, M.D., Ph.D.

The human body lives and functions properly due to metabolism, which represents thousands of biochemical reactions in cells. These reactions are interrelated and are in a state of dynamic equilibrium. In cells of different tissues two kinds of biochemical reactions carried out: one kind provides basic metabolic pathways supported viability of the cells. Another kind of reactions realizes specific for each tissue function. Many functions of different tissues in the organism are controlled by specific division of the brain called **hypothalamus**. The regulation of functional activity by the hypothalamus provides a constancy of the composition of the body's internal medium known as **homeostasis**. Disruption of homeostasis leads to disease development.

External factors, called stressors, can disturb regulatory function of hypothalamus via action on appropriate receptors of central nervous system. These factors can be tentatively divided into physical, chemical and psycho-emotional stressors. High and low ambient temperature, noise, traumas, a severe physical load, starvation, a lack of oxygen, intoxication,

2

different kinds of radiation are all examples of physical and chemical stressors.

The chemical stress factor that is often overlooked is the influence of various chemicals (mainly benzene derivatives) used in building construction as well as the manufacturing of furniture, rugs and plastic goods. Such substances slowly but constantly accumulate inside buildings and then enter the organism via the air we breathe. Chemicals used for the treatment and manufacturing of shoes can be absorbed into the organism through the skin. Despite the fact that such substances enter the organism in very small amounts, their almost constant presence in the blood stream can induce a slight but prolonged state of stress.

Psycho-emotional stressors include intellectual overload, prolonged concentration, lack of sleep, unpleasant events at work or in the family as well as other factors that elicit strong negative emotions. Psycho-emotional stresses frequently accompany physical stresses, thereby increasing their negative influence. The ever-increasing intensity of work and uncertainty of the future are common psycho-emotional stress factors in today's modern society.

The process of re-establishing of homeostasis disturbed by stress is called an **adaptive response**. This process is so named because it enables the organism to adapt to the influence of stressors. **Adaptive response is realized owing to the stress system, which consists of the vegetative nervous system, adrenals, pituitary gland and the hypothalamus—the key component of the system.** Stress signals from the periphery as well as from various brain divisions merge in hypothalamus and activate the stress system. **An activated state of the stress system is what is known as stress.**

The stress system produces various changes in the organism in response to the influence of stress factors, including changes in behavior. The purpose of these changes is to adapt the organism to the changed external conditions. In particular, it helps the organism to overcome difficulties and hazards. It is widely known that under the influence of emotional stress some people have been able to accomplish things that they would never have been able to do in their normal states (such as jumping from a high bridge, lifting a very heavy weight or enduring freezing water). Stress, per the above definition, is not connected only with difficulties and unpleasant events. A state of stress can exist even while experiencing such positive events as making love or watching a sporting event. Stress is a usual reaction of the body to changes in exterior conditions.

CHAPTER TWO
The Consequences of Stress

Light and moderate stress that does not last for a prolonged period of time can have some beneficial effects for humans. A positive stress is a source of optimism, while a light negative stress is a way of training the organism to overcome future difficulties. It is the very strong or the moderate but long-term stress that can lead to pathological changes in the organism. Why does that happen and what mechanisms that are involved?

Despite the great diversity of stressors, the stress system's response reaction to them is virtually uniform or nonspecific. Under the influence of neural impulses, the hypothalamus releases a neuropeptide called corticotropin-releasing hormone. In response to stressors, this hormone interacts with receptors in many brain divisions, producing changes in behavior and stimulating indirectly the excretion of adrenaline and noradrenaline by adrenal medulla. The corticotropin-releasing hormone also enters the pituitary gland, which is connected with hypothalamus and which under the influence of the corticotropin-releasing hormone secretes adrenocorticotropic hormone into the blood stream. This hormone interacts with the adrenal cortex, stimulating the secretion of glucocorticoids (cortisol, cortisone and corticosterone) into the blood stream.

The secretion of adrenaline and noradrenaline into the blood stream is the initial and a short-term reaction of the stress system to the influence of a stressor. These substances produce several effects including a narrowing of capillaries, an elevation of the blood pressure and heart rate, an increase of the blood sugar level, and a reduction of the functional activity of the digestive system.

Unlike adrenaline, glucocorticoids are released later and act significantly longer. They have a broad spectrum of action on cells. In particular, glucocorticoids reduce synthesis of male and female sex hormones, thereby reducing protein synthesis in muscle tissues. This promotes osteoporosis and slower lipid decomposition. They induce a decomposition of muscle proteins, activate glucose synthesis from the decomposed proteins, decrease antioxidant enzyme activity, depress the function of thyroid gland and the activity of immune system.

In addition to a peripheral action, glucocorticoids act via the appropriate receptors in the brain—in particular in the division called **hippocampus** involved in learning and recent memory about stress. Under the influence of glucocorticoids, the hippocampus exerts an inhibiting effect on the stress system, thereby terminating the stress response. Glucocorticoid action on appetite centers in hypothalamus induces changes in appetite. Other brain divisions are also influenced by glucocorticoids.

During short-term but intense stress, when there is a sharp increase in glucocorticoid secretion, the stress system can return the organism to normal without negative consequences. For example, when the world first cosmonaut Yury Gagarin returned from space, his urine glucocorticoid level was 10.7 times higher than normal. A week later, the glucocorticoid content was again back to normal. No deviations in Gagarin's health was detected as a consequence of space flight.

In contrast to short-term stress, a condition of stress which is of long duration, or chronic, does not allow the stress system to return to normal. This can lead to exhaustion of the reserves of the systems involved in the adaptive response which in turn is manifested as various diseases.

Different people react differently to the same stressors depending mostly on inherited peculiarities of the nervous system. Short-term exposure to the same stressor results in a stress that disappears relatively quickly in strong-willed and emotionally stable individuals but which tend to last longer in people with less emotional stability.

The following is an example of differences in stress resistance. Researchers found that usually people who lived next to an airport had an increase in glucocorticoid secretion and changes in electroencephalogram following the loud noise of passing airplanes. The individual reaction to the noise, however, was quite different: thirty-eight percent of people were highly irritated by the sound, twenty-five percent were moderately irritated, ten percent were somewhat irritated, and twenty-seven percent were not irritated at all.

These are the primary symptoms of chronic stress: temporarily impaired functions of the brain, including increased irritability, physical and mental fatigue, inability to concentrate on a particular problem, insomnia, anxiety, a decrease of the reproductive function in men and women.

Prolonged and severe stresses can cause various somatic diseases and functional disturbances in different organs. According to some estimates, prolonged stress is the initial reason for approximately eighty percent of common diseases. The most characteristic illnesses caused by chronic stress include neuroses, depression, common cold, atherosclerosis, cardiovascular diseases, erosive gastritis, ulceration of the stomach and the duodenum, ulcerative colitis, diabetes mellitus, obesity and alcohol abuse.

Psycho-emotional stress most frequently arises during occupational activities. People whose work involves some form of risk or who have high levels of responsibility regularly find themselves in stressful conditions. Soldiers during battle, astronauts, military and civilian pilots, policemen, operators of navigation and surveillance systems, professional athletes, stockbrokers, and managers are among those who usually experience stress. Such occupations demand a particularly well-balanced nervous system. The weaker the person is emotionally, the greater is the risk that he will find himself in a state of chronic stress which in turn can lead to various pathological conditions.

According to statistical data collected in Russia, incidents of cardiovascular diseases due to arteriosclerosis among pilots are up to two-and-a-half times more frequent than in the general population.

Thirty-three percent of navy sailors who worked as radar or acoustic-location system operators developed sleep disorders and other manifestations of stress during sea voyages.

Among Australian air force pilots, fifty seven percent of those decommissioned for medical conditions were as the result of the emotional state of the person. Seventy percent of the pilots in the US strategic air force flying planes with nuclear weapons have been found to suffer from moderate to severe emotional disturbances. Most professional athletes display signs of both physical and emotional stress during preparation and participation in important competitions. The New York Stock Exchange has oxygen dispensers installed on the premises for brokers suffering form ischemic heart attacks.

Although it is difficult to precisely determine the frequency of chronic stress, some estimates indicate that approximately one out of every five Americans experiences emotional stress at work. Marital conflicts are additional social stress factors. Typical stress changes in the organism were studied during thirty-minute marital conflict discussions. Both newlywed couples and older couples, which had been married for four decades, took part in the study. The results showed increased blood pressure, decreased levels of prolactin, increased levels of adrenaline, noradrenaline, growth hormone and adrenocorticotropic hormone, as well as significant repression of immunity. The changes persisted for 24 hours. Women were usually more affected than men during such marital conflicts.

Repeated unresolved marital disagreements may lead to decreased satisfaction with the marriage and chronic stress. Long-term abrasive marital relationship in older couples is often a reason for depression and immunity impairment. The prevalence of chronic stress is evidenced in the fact that more than forty percent of marriages in the US end in divorce.

Although the reasons for psycho-emotional stress are numerous, they often include feelings of insecurity and uncertainty over the future. The American economist Wallace Peterson, in his book "Silent Depression: The Fate of the American Dream", writes: "If you feel you are making and spending more money than you did ten or twenty years ago but are losing ground, if it appears that your children will do less well than you have done, if your job is less secure than it used to be, you are not alone. Millions of other Americans . . . have to run faster to stay in the same place."

People with heightened emotional sensitivity and less self-controlled are more prone to chronic stress for those reasons. Such individuals often respond to stress by overeating or by increasing their alcohol consumption. (Researchers have also noted that those within this group who are more resistant to stress are those who are inclined to overeating, while the less resistant individuals are more prone to alcohol consumption.)

For some time, scientists have tried to understand the causes of overweight problem and increased alcohol consumption. In the United States, for example, it is especially worrisome that the number of people who are significantly overweight has increased steadily. Over the last twenty years, the increase is over thirty percent. This trend is expected to continue in the future.

Beside genetic factor, the correlation between stress and problem of overweight points out the ineffectiveness of various diets to solve the problem. Similarly, the case can be made that there is a causal relationship between low resistance to stress and increased alcohol consumption.

One of the early and important consequences of chronic stress is the decrease of the functional activity of the immune system. This can reduce the resistance to various infections, inflammatory lung disorders, allergies, asthma, autoimmune diseases, ulcerative colitis, rheumatoid arthritis, and the decrease in the body's ability to repair tissue damaged by mechanical, thermal, radiation and chemical factors.

Chronic stress aggravates already existing diabetes mellitus of both types. Heightened levels of glucocorticoids in the blood during stress can produce an insulin resistance, leading to hyperglycemia, hyperholesterolemia and obesity.

Premenopausal and postmenopausal women are less resistant to emotional stressors than women whose estrogen activity has not changed. The lack of adaptation is more typical of postmenopausal women.

Estrogen treatment further lowers their stress-induced response.

During chronic stress, the activity of peroxidase, an enzyme that decomposes endogenous H_2O_2, decreases. Hydrogen peroxide is formed as a by-product of normal energy metabolism. Strenuous physical activities and sports cause a dramatic increase in oxygen uptake by muscles and other tissues. Hydrogen peroxide is reactive oxygen specie that can interact with cellular membranes and DNA, disrupting the functions of many tissues and trigger the development of cancer. Specialized antioxidant mechanisms are designed to protect cells from such oxidative damages. One of these is the decomposition of H_2O_2 by peroxidase, the enzyme activity of which is repressed during stress.

It is interesting to note that in fruit fly Drosophila mutation of one of the genes (mth) increases stress resistance and simultaneously increases life span by thirty-five percents. Scientists studying the influence of stress in man at the cellular level concluded that stress accelerates the aging processes and that the organism becomes less resistant to stress due to the weakened defense systems and energy metabolism with age. Stimulation of energy metabolism and defense-repair systems in the body may therefore increase the life span of the organism.

Part II: The Promoters of Nonspecific Resistance of the Organism.

CHAPTER THREE
What Are Adaptogens?

In accordance with Hans Selye's theory the response to stress is so- called "general adaptation syndrome". The term "adaptogen" derives from the "general adaptation syndrome". It was introduced into the scientific literature in 1947 by the Russian scientist N. Lasarev to designate **a substance of plant origin that is able to increase the nonspecific resistance of the organism to the effects of various stressors and thereby to promote adaptation of the body to stressful conditions.** Although the specific mechanisms of action of adaptogens are diverse and not all of them are clear, we do know that their activity is predominantly directed to the maintenance of homeostasis in the organism.

In the course of evolution, animals and humans have used plants as a major source of nutrients. Their metabolism therefore evolved as a consequence of this. As a result, activation of many metabolic reactions in the human organism requires plant-derived substances, such as vitamins.

As various other non-vitamin plant substances were studied in more detail, it became clear that some of them are also capable to activate the cellular metabolism and functionality of various systems of the body.

Besides fruits and vegetables, humans have since ancient times used specific plants in the form of spices, condiments, tinctures, and teas to elevate appetite, mood, and to aid in restoring physical and mental fitness. Some of those plants were used by healers of the past as medicines to counter fatigue, for increase of sexual function and to elevate the general physical tone in older people. Scientific research has now confirmed adaptogenic properties of the plants but for centuries, generations of healers have selected such plants by carefully observing their effects on thousands of people.

From the point of view of modern pharmacology, such processes of selecting physiologically active natural substances may appear primitive. This is, however, an arrogant view—an overestimation of final efficacy of most modern man-made drugs. In particular, artificial substance can hardly serve as prophylactic remedy against common diseases and functional disorders. Some drugs effectively relieve illness symptoms, but they may be used only for a short period of time and can't be used for prophylactic purposes.

The probability that an artificial compound is able to harmlessly integrate into the intricate mechanisms of homeostasis regulation—processes that have been fine-tuned by evolution over millennia—is very low, at least at the levels of current human knowledge. Additionally, the most convincing method to demonstrate the effectiveness of a drug and its level of toxicity is to use humans as trial subjects. That is exactly the approach used by those healers from the past.

Laboratory and clinical studies of plants that possess adaptogenic properties were began in Russia in the middle of past age. Historical data about "healing" plants from the mountains of Altay, in the southeastern regions of Siberia and Far East formed the basis for these studies. Expeditions staffed with botany experts went to those distant locations and brought back plant samples. These were then used for the first scientific studies to understand the influence of the plants on the human organism.

The researches documented how various preparations produced from these adaptogenic plants influenced the human body. Since it had become clear that adaptogens are effectively extracted from the plants by ethyl alcohol, the researchers used in their work primarily ethanol plant extracts.

The adaptogenenic plants have characteristic spectra of effects that may, nevertheless, partly overlap. Action spectrum of each plant is determined by the molecular structure of the adaptogens, which are the constituents of a particular plant. A magnitude of physiological effects of the adaptogens

depends on their concentration in the blood stream, the deepness of stress-induced deterioration of homeostasis and readiness of the target-cell receptors to interact with the adaptogens.

When present in the blood of a healthy organism, adaptogens serve as regulatory buffers, ready to restore homeostasis as soon as it is disturbed.

The important difference between adaptogens and various stimulators is the ability of adaptogens to return to norm biochemical processes, which have been disturbed by stress. Adaptogens do not influence processes that are normal. Unlike adaptogens, natural stimulators such as caffeine, nicotine, cocaine, and cardiac glycosides, act with no regard to the state of homeostasis and they exert their influence on biochemical processes whether normal or not.

Not all adaptogens have yet been identified. Identification of adaptogens faces many difficulties primarily because isolated substances of a particular plant often do not have adaptogenic properties or properties that are rather weak. The adaptogenic activity of a plant depends greatly on the cooperative and synergic effects of several substances. Some isolated substances do, however, show an adaptogenic action that has made their identification possible. It is important to note that the action spectrum of an isolated adaptogen is usually narrower compared than a whole extract prepared from the same plant.

The adaptogenic properties of the plants that have undergone the most careful and rigorous testing by Russian scientists and physicians are described in the following chapters. Over the course of many years, medical doctors have tested and employed extracts from these plants. The adaptogenic extracts have therefore been included in the Russian Pharmacopoeia and are recommended for patients in hospitals, outpatients and for practically healthy people in everyday life as the remedies restored some functional upsets, physical and psychical fatigue and as prophylactic remedies increased a nonspecific resistance of the organism.

CHAPTER FOUR
Rhodiola rosea

Rhodiola rosea is a perennial grassy plant that belongs to the *Grassulaceae* family. It is also known by the common name "Golden root". Rhodiola is a rather polymorph plant whose anatomical structure and content of biologically active compounds can vary from region to region. In Russia, Rhodiola grows in mountainous areas within the polar circle, in the mountains of southern Siberia (Altay, Sayani, and Tuva) as well as on Sakhalin island and Kamchatka. The plant regenerates very slowly (eight to ten years). The collection of wild Rhodiola is, therefore, strictly limited.

The roots of Rhodiola rosea have an unusual reddish golden color. The plant, however, was not given the name Golden Root simply because of its root color. It has long been a highly valued plant because of its ability to restore strength and to preserve health. On his wedding day, the Siberian groom traditionally received Golden Root as a sexual stimulator. Chinese emperors sent expeditions to the mountains of Altay to search for the plant while local inhabitants tried to keep the locations of the plant secret. Golden Root was frequently smuggled into China as a highly valuable commodity: Scientific studies on Golden Root began in Russia in the 1960's after botanists had identified it in the mountain forests of Altay as Rhodiola rosea. Different groups of substances have since been detected in the ethanol extract from its roots: tannins, sterols, glycosides, flavonoids, organic acids, anthraglycosides, essential oils, waxes, and tertiary alcohols. Among these groups were identified, in particular, these compounds: salidrosid, keampferol, p-tyrosol, betaphenylethylacetate, phenylethanol, beta-phenylacetate, cinnamaldehyde, gallic acid, oxalate, citrate, malate, succinate. Not all compounds have yet been identified.

We do not know precisely how each of these constituents contributes to the physiological effects of Rhodiola extract. It appears, however, that one of them possesses most of the physiological activity characteristic of the plant. It was isolated, crystallized and identified as a glycoside called **salidrosid**. Its content in Rhodiola root is approximately 0.2%. The aglicone part of its molecule is structurally close to dihydroxyphenylalanine (dopa), a precursor of catecholaminergic neurotransmitters. It has been experimentally demonstrated that salidrosid activates the transmission of nerve impulses in catecholaminergic synapses of the brain. However, the action spectrum of salidrosid only partly coincides with the action spectrum of whole extract from Rhodiola. Physiological effectiveness of isolated salidrosid is about thirty times less than that of the whole extract.

Animal testing shows that during prolonged physical work, Rhodiola extract increases the adaptation to exhaustion by more than a factor of two. During physical fatigue, the extract stimulates in muscles the synthesis of adenosine triphosphate (ATP)—a main source of energy in any cell; increases the rate of lipolysis and results in an earlier mobilization of lipids from adipose tissues; increases glycogen concentration in muscles, liver, and brain.

Rhodiola extract increases activity of the cytochrome system and some other oxidative enzymes. It also prevents a reduction of tissue concentrations of glutamic and aspartic acids that play important roles in muscle protein metabolism. Structural changes of mitochondrial membranes in muscle fibers under physical stress, as detected by electron microscopy, are significantly less pronounced when Rhodiola extract was used prior to exercise.

During physical stress, the energy supplied to the brain decreases. Concentrations of ATP, creatine phosphate and glycogen in brain tissues drop. The introduction of Rhodiola extract before exercise maintains almost the initial levels of those compounds, thereby sustaining the energy supply to the brain. This is most likely the result of an intensification of oxidative phosphorylation processes under the influence of the extract.

Human clinical trials show that Rhodiola extract increases the endurance to physical stress by twelve percent. The resistance to repeated physical stress in an organism already fatigued increases by twenty-eight percents. The extract also had a positive effect on some functional parameters including a normalization of blood pressure and pulse rate after heavy physical stress.

Rhodiola extract has an anti-toxic effect against many chemical compounds (e.g. strychnine and aniline). Since aniline causes production of metahemoglobin that decreases tissue oxygen supply, the effect of Rhodiola on hypoxia has been studied. Administration of the extract to mice prior to experiments significantly increased their life span in an airtight vessel, indicating an increased resistance to hypoxia. The antihypoxic action of Rhodiola has likewise been registered by oxyhemography in man under prolonged and intensive physical stress.

It is interesting to note that Rhodiola extract also have antihypnotic and antianesthetic properties. Administration of the extract reduced the duration of sleep caused by hexobarbital and barbital in mice to fifty-four and sixty-two percent respectively compared to mice not treated with the extract. Pretreatment of mice with 0.1 ml of Rhodiola extract once a day for ten days increased lethal dose (LD 50) of 40% ethyl alcohol from 24.1 to 56.2 ml per kilogram of body weight—the extract increased resistance to toxic effects of alcohol by more than a factor of two.

Rhodiola extract increases the ability to perform intellectual work for prolonged periods of time, especially if such work requires a high degree of concentration. Studies on two groups of 117 students (male and female 20 to 28 years of age) using a specially designed "correction" test assessed the intellectual abilities both qualitatively and quantitatively based on speed and quantity of corrected characters. Following one dose of 0.5 ml of Rhodiola extract mistakes dropped by four percent (statistically true value). The number of corrected characters were by six percent lower among the students who received Rhodiola supplementation compared to the control students.

Rhodiola extract prevents a drop in intellectual capabilities due to alcohol. Twelve men (20-28 years old) in one group took 100 ml 40% alcohol while men in another group took 100 ml of alcohol supplemented with 0.5 ml of Rhodiola extract. An assessment of the subject's intellectual state was done one hour after the alcohol consumption using the same "correction" test mentioned above. In the control group, the number of corrected characters did not change but the number of mistakes increased by seventy-seven percents. Among the students who received Rhodiola supplementation, the speed remained the same, but the number of errors increased by only fifteen percents under the influence of the alcohol.

Rhodiola extract produces some short-term hypoglycemia in animals that have normal blood sugar level, reducing the sugar concentration by ten to fifteen percent. Human clinical trials on diabetic patients have shown no significant hypoglycemic effect when the extract was taken orally. The extract did, however, effectively prevent the development of hypoglycemia in rabbits injected with insulin. Insulin administration reduced mean blood sugar level from 104 mg/100 ml to 46 mg/100 ml in control animals. While under prophylactic oral administration of Rhodiola extract (15 minutes before the insulin injection), blood sugar level never fell below 84 mg/100 ml.

Prophylactic oral administration of the extract also prevents the development of hyperglycemia. Injection of adrenaline produced an average increase in blood sugar content by fifty percents while pretreatment with Rhodiola extract reduced this response to only seventeen percents.

As can be seen from this, Rhodiola extract does not show curative effect on already existing processes that cause diabetes. But it does prevent the development of both hypo– and hyperglycemias when taken prophylactically. In other words, it maintains the normal state independently of the direction that deviation from the norm.

Rhodiola extract similarly affects blood cell count. It also prevents development of leukocytosis and leukopenia, as well as erythrocytosis and erythropenia in experimental rabbits. **This ability to maintain the normal function of a particular body system irrespective of the direction of the deviation from the norm is characteristic of adaptogens.** In animals whose pituitary gland had been surgically removed, a protective action of Rhodiola extract against leukocytosis is not detected.

In animals, Rhodiola extract demonstrates some anti-cancer activity. The extract was administered with food to a highly tumorogenic mice line starting at the age of two months. Among the control group, the first tumors (breast adenocarcinoma) appeared at the age of eight months, while the group treated with the extract developed first tumors only at the age of eleven months. The frequency of tumor formation in the group treated with Rhodiola extract was three times lower than that of the control group. Rhodiola extract also reduces the toxicity caused by cancer chemotherapy drugs: fewer pronounced changes were noted in the peripheral blood and cells of the intestinal walls.

Under mental fatigue Rhodiola extract promotes restoration of central nervous system activity. Rise of electrical activity of brain cortex following administration of Rhodiola extract has been observed by electroencephalography. Changed electrical patterns produced with Rhodiola extract are very similar to those caused by Leuzea extract.

They differ significantly from the pattern changes produced by the well-known psychostimulator amphetamine. As a result supplementation with Rhodiola extract, attention span and concentration improved, psychomotor reaction accelerated and the immediate memorization improved. These effects were the more noticeable the more mental fatigue was pronounced.

Numerous human clinical trials have validated the effectiveness of Rhodiola extract against the following pathological states: asthenia, neuroses, hypotension, decreased sexual potency, secondary amenorrhea and hearing impairment.

The state of asthenia often develops in otherwise healthy people from prolonged and intense intellectual work. Asthenia is characterized by decreased ability to perform work, slow comprehension, inability to concentrate and attention deficit, headache, and sleeplessness. Emotional instability, inability to tolerate loud sounds, bright light and other irritants are also frequently observed. People who prophylactically took Rhodiola extract several days before the beginning a period consisting of intensive mental work and then continued to use the herb during the entire period, did not develop signs of asthenia. Signs of asthenia had earlier been evident among the same group of people doing similar work but when they had not received Rhodiola treatment. Rhodiola extract has been proven to be an effective medicine in eighty percent of patients with functional asthenia, including people recovering from infectious and somatic diseases.

Anxiety disorders usually occur as a result of chronic stress. Other usual symptoms of such stress-induced conditions include sleep disorders, bad mood, hypotension, uncomfortable feelings in the heart region, and gastritis. As a result of Rhodiola extract intake these manifestations were significantly milder or disappeared completely depending on their initial severity.

One of the common manifestations of such stress-induced conditions in men is weak erection, premature ejaculation or combination of both. Thirty five men with sexual function problems were subjects in a study using Rhodiola extract in the course of three months. A significant correction of the sexual function was observed in twenty six of the men. Improvement of the composition of prostate gland excreta was also noted.

Under chronic stress and some other conditions, hypogonadotropic or secondary amenorrhea can arise in women. Treatment of thirty three women suffering from secondary amenorrhea were treated with Rhodiola extract for twenty to forty days, resulted in the restoration of menstrual function in twenty five women. Eleven women were able to become pregnant.

Intensive and prolonged exposure to noise is a powerful physical stressor that can cause some degree of hearing loss. The effects of Rhodiola extract on people with impaired hearing was studied on a group that included three pilots and nineteen construction workers who were subjected to noise levels of 100 to 180 decibel during a working day.

Two weeks after treatment with Rhodiola extract, twenty people showed improvement in air and bone speech sound conductivity by 10 to 20 decibel, while two had a 20 to 30 decibel improvement. High-frequency sound air conductivity increased by 10 decibel in nine people, by 30 to 40 decibel in three individuals, and did not change in ten people.

It is also worth noting that in the majority of patients, treatment with Rhodiola extract results in an improvement of general physical and mental state irrespective of the nature of the pathology.

CHAPTER FIVE
Leuzea carthamoides

Leuzea carthamoides (also called *Rhaponticum carthamoides*) is a rare endemic plant belonging to the *Compositae* family. It is a big herbal perennial plant, reaching 180 cm in height. Leuzea grows on the mountain slopes in a limited area of southern Siberia (Altay, Sayani); it does not exist as a wild-growing plant in other regions of the world. Because of the limited distribution of Leuzea in nature and because the plant grows slowly, the collection of wild-growing Leuzea in Russia is under government control and is severely restricted.

The history of Leuzea as a medicinal plant began in ages past when local hunters noticed the unusual behavior of a variety of deer known as Maral. At the time of mating, when males fight each other and need to restore their strength, stags dig out and eat Leuzea roots. Local healers discovered that consumption of dried Leuzea roots by man also helped him recover from fatigue and increase his sexual potency. The plant was thereafter named "Maral root", now the official common name of Leuzea.

Scientific studies of Leuzea's influence on the organism began in Russia in the 1940's, during World War II, when the country had a needed medication to help restore the strength and stamina of its soldiers. From these studies came the discoveries that an ethanol extract of dried Leuzea roots contain tannins, phytoecdysones, flavonols, glycosides, lignins, alkaloids, vitamins, organic acids, and some yet-to-be-identified compounds.

Numerous experiments on animals and human clinical trials have made it possible to establish that Leuzea root extract:

- Increases the rate at which ATP (source of energy in cells) is restored;

- Contributes to an increase of muscle mass;
- Reinforces contractions of the heart muscle;
- Improves blood circulation in muscles and brain;
- Increases resistance to oxygen starvation;
- Elevates the viability and mobility of spermatozoids in vitro;
- Accelerates sexual maturity and the first pregnancy of female animals;
- Prevents development of experimental hyper- and hypoglycemia, leukocytosis, leukopenia, erythrocytosis and erythropenia;
- Improves transmission of impulses in interneuronal synapses depressed by the hypnotic drug sodium barbital;
- Neutralizes the suppressive effect on the brain by sodium barbital;
- Restores the capacity to focus, concentrate and perform mental work in humans while mentally fatigued;
- Increases the resistance to the common cold.

In addition, clinical trials have shown that Leuzea extract has the capability to prevent and eliminate stress-induced pathological conditions, especially during their initial stages. In particular, it improves the focus and attention in persons whose duties require great concentration (such as air traffic controllers, pilots). Leuzea extract prevents stress-induced sleep disorders and does not evoke any unpleasant sensations, such as psycho-emotional retardation, sluggishness, apathy and headaches, which were observed following the intake of sleeping pills. The extract has a positive influence on the initial stages asthenia and sexual malfunction. It also slightly decreases the sugar content in the blood during the initial stage of diabetes mellitus.

Among various active constituents of Leuzea extract, the most interesting is **ecdysterone**—a polyhydroxylated sterol belonging to ecdysone group. The ecdysterone content in dried Leuzea roots can reach as high as 0.5%. Ecdysterone also exists in some insects and crustaceans but not in vertebrate animals or in humans. In insects and crustaceans, ecdysterone is synthesized in trace quantities as a hormone to regulate protein synthesis.

Because ecdysterone was not known to exist in humans, scientists at first did not pay attention to man as subject for research of ecdysterone activity. Later, scientists established that ecdysterone is physiologically active with respect to mammalian and human cells. It has now been demonstrated that ecdysterone:

- Possesses anabolic activity—the ability to increase muscle mass—while not disturbing the androgen function (in contrast to well known anabolic steroids);
- Activates synthesis of glutamate decarboxylase (an enzyme which is responsible for synthesis of gamma-aminobutyric acid, an inhibitory neurotransmitter in the brain);
- Activates the brain synthesis of acetylcholine esterase (an enzyme which participates in regulation of nerve impulse transmission in cholinergic neurons);
- Activates synthesis of dopa decarboxylase (an enzyme participating in formation of adrenaline);
- Activates synthesis of catalase (an enzyme that destroys harmful H_2O_2);
- Activates synthesis of glucose dehydrogenase, acid phosphatase and malate dehydrogenase (enzymes which take part in energy providing of the cell);
- Protects nuclear chromatin (a chromosome component) in liver cells against free radical oxidation induced by tetrachloromethane in experimental animals, thus significantly increasing their survival;
- Provides protective action against experimental atherosclerosis in rabbits;
- Restores phospholipids of liver mitochondria pathologically changed by insulin insufficiency under experimental alloxan diabetes mellitus in animals;

- Eliminates experimental arrhythmia and improves heart contractility during coronary artery occlusion in animals;
- Possesses an immunomodulating effect on lymphocyte production by spleen.

The mechanism of ecdysterone action is probably similar to that of human steroid hormones. This means that steroid hormone receptors of human cells interact with the ecdysterone. Human endogenous hormones have, however, an advantage over ecdysterone because of their higher affinity to the hormone receptors. When human steroid hormones are produced in sufficient quantities in the body, ecdysterone can't compete with endogenous hormones for the receptors and therefore does not evoke an effect. But when there is a deficiency in the body of its own hormones, ecdysterone can bind to unoccupied steroid hormone receptors, replacing the missing endogenous hormone.

During the human organism's adaptive response to stress factors, the role of ecdysterone consists primarily of the activation of a synthesis of various proteins. For instance, repeated physical stress of muscles triggers an adaptive synthesis of oxidative enzymes, contractile proteins in muscle cells and the growth of new muscle capillaries. This occurs with the participation of testosterone—it is this hormone, which activates the genes controlling protein synthesis. During exhaustive physical exercise, the testosterone concentration in the blood stream drops. Ecdysterone can then become an effective substitute for the missing testosterone, displaying its anabolic activity and promoting the adaptation to physical stress.

Leuzea extract contains also biologically active compounds other than ecdysterone. In particular, there are some flavonols, such as **kaempferol**, which are well known active components of non-enzymatic antioxidant system in cells. But perhaps less well known is the fact that kaempferol possesses also estrogenic activity. Ecdysterone has higher affinity to testosterone receptors, while kaempferol binds more readily to estrogen receptors. The affinity of kaempferol to estrogen receptors is one tenth of that of endogenous estrogens.

Based on existing data, it may appear that the majority of the effects caused by Leuzea extract are determined by interaction of some Leuzea constituents with the receptors of human steroid hormones. Thus, the constituents play a role of low affinity hormonal buffer in the body. Anti-oxidant capability of some flavonoids also contributes to the adaptogenic effects. More detailed mechanisms of biological activity of Leuzea compounds have to be the subject of future researches.

CHAPTER FIVE
Eleutherococcus senticosus

Eleutherococcus senticosus is known also as "Siberian Ginseng" because its influence on the human organism is to some extent similar to that of the well-known Chinese Panax Ginseng. Both of these plants belong to *Araliaceae* family. This is, however, the only thing that they have in common—they are two completely different plants. Eleutherococcus is a perennial bush with highly developed branching root system that can reach from 2 to 5 m in height, while Panax Ginseng is a comparatively small herb with a thin trunk and a rod-like root. Eleutherococcus grows in the Far East area of Russia as well as in northeastern China, northern Korea and in Japan.

The adaptogenic properties of Eleutherococcus were first discovered in 1965 and extensively studied in pharmacological laboratory of Dr. I. Brekhman at the Far East Center of the Russian Academy of Sciences in Vladivostok. The physiological action of Eleutherococcus extract is determined predominantly by the presence of six different glycosides called **eleutherosides,** aglycones of which differ from one another. Individual eleutherosides isolated from the extract and their mixture are, however, less biologically active than the extract as a whole.

Primary scientific studies of Eleutherococcus as adaptogenic plant have been published in Russia. Several articles also published in international journals. The various biological effects of Eleutherococcus root extract have been summarized in the books by B. Kamen and D. B. Mowrey (see Bibliography). The majority of laboratory and clinical tests show that the plant's effects are partially similar to those described for Rhodiola and Leuzea. I will, therefore, describe here only those effects that I consider most significant.

A large number of experiments on animals and humans have shown that Eleutherococcus extract increases the capacity to perform physical work and accelerates the recovery after intense work. These effects are based on an activation of the oxygen supply necessary for energy generation in cells as well as on the ability of Eleutherococcus to modulate the activity of some endocrine glands. This property of Eleutherococcus is especially valuable for athletes.

Prophylactic treatment with Eleutherococcus reduces the toxicity of some harmful chemicals and normalizes leukocyte count in the blood. Tests show, however, that these effects are lower in Eleutherococcus than in Rhodiola.

Large-scale human studies with people whose work involved a high degree of concentration over a long period under psychologically stressful conditions, established that Eleutherococcus extract reduced psychological fatigue and accelerated recovery during rest. This anti-stress property of Eleutherococcus has been beneficial to Russian cosmonauts during long expeditions into space.

Eleutherococcus extract has an ability to modulate the activity of the human immune system. Taking Eleutherococcus extract three times a day for a period of four weeks increases the number of immunocompetent lymphocytes and immunoglobulins in the blood. Eleutherococcus extract increases in vitro phagocytosis of yeast by granulocytes and monocytes from healthy donors by thirty to forty-five percent. Eleutherococcus promotes an increase in the interferon production in response to viral infections, improving the resistance of the human organism against viruses.

A regular prophylactic intake of Eleutherococcus during one year by one thousand miners living and working under adverse climate conditions of extreme northern region of Russia (in the city of Norilsk) drastically reduced the frequency of common cold sickness.

During a long sea voyage in tropical areas, navy seamen displayed a spectrum of different functional imbalances characteristic of stress. This resulted in a reduced ability to work and caused a worsening of overall health, specifically a decreased resistance to infections.

Studies done on seventy-seven sailors showed that treatment with Eleutherococcus commencing at the very beginning of a voyage and continuing for thirty days completely or partially prevented deviations from the norm in seventy to seventy-five percent of the sailors.

Animal experiments together with observations made on cancer patients have demonstrated a positive effect of Eleutherococcus extract during chemo- and radiotherapy. Improvements during rehabilitation after surgical tumor removal were also observed.

Eleutherococcus extract decreases ultrastructural lesions in the ischemic area during experimental myocardial infarction in animals and improves heart tissue regeneration.

Researchers have noted an increased resistance to changes of ambient temperature, oxygen deprivation, as well as an improvement in the general state of patients with some common diseases under the influence of Eleutherococcus extract.

CHAPTER SIX
Schizandra chinensis

Schizandra chinensis, one of the members of the *Schizandraceae* family, is a perennial wood-like liana. It grows in the easternmost regions of Siberia, in China, Japan, and Korea and in some other regions.

Roots, stems and leaves of Schizandra have a strong lemony smell, which is why the plant is known in Russia as a lemon tree. In China it is called "Wu-wei-zi"; in Japan Schizandra has the name "Hoku-gomishi" or "Kita-gomishi".

Schizandra is a traditional medicine in China since ancient times. Inhabitants in those regions of Siberia where the plant grows have used its fruits for centuries to provide strength. The berries are also a traditional source of juice, while the liana bark and leaves are tea substitutes. Scientific studies of Schizandra began in Russia in the 1940's. Essential fatty oils, tannins, various organic acid, vitamins, sugars, flavonoids, lignans, sesquiterpenoids and other compounds were identified in the Schizandra berries. Alcohol extracts from fruits and seeds possess most of the plants physiological activity. Therefore, such extracts have been the ones mostly used in clinical trials.

The first compound that has adaptogenic properties characteristic to Schizandra was isolated in 1951. Russian scientists mapped its molecular structure in 1962. This compound is called **schizandrin** and turned out to be a lignan with a dibenzocyclooctadiene skeleton. Five other compounds with spectral properties similar to those of schizandrin have also been detected. Japanese scientists, who studied the structures of these compounds in 1979, called them gomisin A, B, C, F, G. Their structural skeleton is also based on dibenzocyclooctadiene.

Like schizandrin, gomisin A, B, and C also possess biological activity. However, similar to other adaptogenic plants, the whole extract from Schizandra fruits have a broader spectrum of activity compared to that of isolated compounds. Although there are some suppositions concerning mechanisms of physiological action of Schizandra fruits compounds the mechanisms are still the subject of future study.

Animal testing shows that both Schizandra extract and schizandrin have a positive effect on the functioning of the central nervous system. This includes a reduction of spinal reflex times. Electroencephalogram analyses have demonstrated that schizandrin can eliminate an inhibition of the brain's electric activity caused by chloral hydrate, amobarbital and chlorpromazine. Some experimental data indicate that Schizandra lignans can act as modulators of function of catecholaminergic synapses.

During physical stress, Schizandra extract increases oxygen supply to tissues, in particular to brain tissues but also to a lesser degree to muscles and liver. Researchers have also noted that Schizandra extract increases the activity of some enzymes that take part in oxidative phosphorylation.

Prophylactic use of Schizandra significantly impedes the development of experimental arteriosclerosis in rabbits and dogs fed large amounts of cholesterol.

Shizandra fruits extract is used in Korea for the treatment of cardiovascular symptoms associated especially with menopausal symptoms. Recently it has been shown that the extract acts as a week fytoestrogen. Some schizandrins are platelet-activating factor (PAF) antagonists, which makes it possible for them to act as modulators of vascular tone.

In carbon tetrachloride (CCl_4) poisoned mice Schizandrins enhance liver mitochondrial glutathione status, which decreases the hepatotoxic effect of CCl_4. Animal testing has demonstrated that gomisin A inhibits the development of preneoplastic lesions in liver and skin from some carcinogens. Some schizandrins have a strong scavenging effect on active oxygen radicals—its scavenging effect on hydroxyl radicals, for example, is greater than that of vitamins E and C.

Prophylactic treatment with Schizandra extract reduces fatigue and improves the results of runners competing in medium and long distance events but such treatment has no effects on sprinters who run 100-meter races.

The effects of Schizandra extract and schizandrins on the ability to concentrate an attention was studied on telegraph operators working two to five hours at maximum speed. Taking Schizandra extracts did not significantly change the rate of typing but reduced the average number of errors reduced by a factor of 1.5 to 2.

Many tests have showed that intake of Schizandra extract improves night vision, increases sensitivity of the eyes to red light, accelerates adaptation to darkness and improves sight by 0.2-0.3 D in the majority of those studied. This property of Schizandra together with its effects of enhancing concentration has proven very useful to drivers, especially for older people since the ability of eyes to adapt to darkness decreases with age—older drivers are more likely to be blinded by headlights from oncoming traffic.

Preventive effects against the common cold have been documented as a result of the prophylactic use of Schizandra extract for a period of twenty-two days. Three groups of people participated in this study:

children from one to seven years old (270 people), students (559 people) and adults (700 people). The adults received 1.0 ml of Schizandra extract a day while children were given extract in juice based on their weight. The average frequency of common cold among the three groups taking Schizandra (758 people) was forty three percents lower than that of the control groups (771 people).

CONCLUSION

Particular feature of adaptogenic effects of the four plants extracts are determined by some factors: the molecular structure of adaptogenic substances, the extent of the adaptogen's affinity to certain cellular receptors and concentration of the adaptogens in the extract.

From the description of physiological effects of the plants it seems like their action spectra are partially overlapped. However that impression can be not correct. The seeming overlapping is probably the consequence of no precise methodology that doesn't permit to reveal existing differences in the effects of different plant extracts. One type of immune system cells (of bone marrow, for instance) can interact with the adaptogen from one plant while other immune system cells (of spleen) can interact with the adaptogen from another plant, but both adaptogens can evoke general effect - activation of immune response. Analogically, cells of different divisions of central nervous system also have different membrane receptors and can interact with different adaptogens. As a result, two different adaptogens can evoke activation of central nervous system that is registered as restoration of mental workability. Registration of more specific biochemical changes in immune and central nervous systems could reveal the differences between effects of the two adaptogens.

With the aim of utilization of whole action spectrum of the extracts from Leuzea, Rhodiola, Eleutherococcus and Schizandra, the adaptogenic preparation "AdMax" has been recently manufactured by NULAB Inc., Clearwater, FL. The preparation is a combination of dry extracts from the four plants. Clinical observations suggest, in particular, that the preparation restores the suppressed immunity and mitigates side effects of chemotherapy in ovarian cancer patients.

As mentioned earlier, some compounds of adaptogenic plants (such as phytoecdysones and flavonols) can bind to steroid hormone receptors of different cells, including cells of the brain. The relative binding affinities of these compounds to some cellular receptors is 10 to 100 times lower than that of human hormones. This is why these plant compounds interact with the receptors primarily when there is a deficiency in the endogenous hormones. Thereby they play a role of low affinity hormonal buffer in the blood during stress when the quantity of steroid hormones drops in the blood stream. **A restoration of the hormonal balance in the body is, probably, most important mechanism to restore homeostasis disturbed by stress.**

The compounds possessed antioxidant properties also make contribution to adaptogenic effects. Some other, even minor, compounds are important because they can act either independently or as co-effectors for other compounds, thereby promoting synergic effect of the extract constituents. So, **adaptogenic properties of the plants are determined by cooperative and**

synergic action of a number of their constituents. The isolation of individual compounds from the extracts essentially results in a drug that does not possess the complete action spectrum characteristic of the plant, which it came from.

The effectiveness of adaptogen's action in the most part depends on physiological state of the human body and individual emotional sensitivity. In general, the more functional deviation from normal, the stronger adaptogenic effect. Adaptogens usually have no effect on the normal functioning of the organism.

Disturbance of homeostasis by stress is the primary stage of functional upsets and sickness development. It is why the restoration of homeostasis by adaptogens prevents some sicknesses. This is the fundamental difference between adaptogens and typical pharmaceutical drugs, which is directed to symptom elimination of an already raised disease. With some exceptions, adaptogens have reduced effects on an already developed disease and in this case their role lies mostly in the prevention of complications to the disease and in a strengthening of general state of the organism.

Numerous studies have showed no significant side effects during long-term oral intake of the extracts at normal doses. Some persons do have, however, an increased sensitivity to the plant extracts and they mark, in particular, insomnia if they take of the extract in a second part of the day. The persons who are under medical care especially for cardiovascular and neurological diseases should consult their physicians concerning intake of the extracts.

The pharmaceutical paradigm: one drug—one symptom is widely spread. Exactly like this most pharmaceutical drugs act. In contrast to that, action of adaptogens doesn't direct to elimination of the symptoms of already existing diseases. Adaptogen action is directed to restoration of stress-induced disturbance of homeostasis in the organism. Thereby it restores functional activity and promotes nonspecific resistance of the body against sicknesses. It is why adaptogens possess much broader spectrum of action than most pharmaceutical drugs.

BIBLIOGRAPHY

Abidov, M. et al. 2003. Effects of extracts from Rhodiola rosea and Rhodiola crenulata (Crassulaceae) roots on ATP content in mitochondria of skeletal muscles. Bull. Exp. Biol. Med. 136: 585. (Russian)

Afanasieva, T.N. & N.P. Lebkova. 1987. Effect of Eleutherococcus on the subcellular structures of the heart in experimental myocardial infarct. Bull. Exp. Biol. Med. 103: 212. (Russian)

Antoshechkin, A.G. 2001. On intracellular formation of ethanol and its possible role in energy metabolism. Alcohol Alcohol. 36: 608.

Aragona, M. et al. 1996. Lymphocyte number and stress parameter modifications in untreated breast cancer patients with depressive mood and previous life stress. J. Exp. Ther. Oncol. 1: 354.

Baltayev, U.A. et al. 1997. 24(24(1))[Z]-dehydroamarasterone B, a phytoecdysteroid from seeds of Leuzea carthamoides. Phytochemistry 46: 103.

Bespalov, V.G. et al. 1992. The inhibiting effect of phytoadaptogenic preparations from bioginseng, Eleutherococcus senticosus and Rhaponticum carthamoides on the development of nervous system tumors in rats induced by N-nitrosoethylurea. Vopr. Onkol. 38: 1073. (Russian)

Blagojeviae, M. et al. 1996. The relationship between stress resistance and stress recovery speed with the indicators of compensated and decompensated fatigue. In: Sports Psychology: New Trends and Applications. Y. Theodorakis & A. Papaioannou, Eds. International Congress on Sport Psychology. Komotini, Greece. p. 309.

Bocharova, O.A. 1999. Adaptogens as agents for prophylactic oncology. Vestn. Ross. Akad. Med. Nauk 5: 49. (Russian)

Bohn, B., C.T. Nebe & C. Birr. 1987. Flow-cytometric studies with eleutherococcus extract as an immunomodulatory agent. Arzneimittelforschung 37: 1193.

Bol'shakova, I.V., E.L. Lozovskaia & I.I. Sapezhinskii. 1997. Antioxidant properties of a series of extracts from medicinal plants. Biofizika 42: 480. (Russian)

Boon-Niermeijer, E.K. et al. 2000. Phyto-adaptogens protect against environmental stress-induced death of embryos from the freshwater snail Lymnaea stagnalis. Phytomedicine 7: 389.

Bradbury, T.N. & B. Karney. 1991. Longitudinal study of marital interaction and dysfunction: Review and analysis. Clin. Psychol. Rev. 13: 15.

Brekhman, I.I. & O.I. Kirillov. 1969. Effect of eleutherococcus on alarm-phase of stress. Life Sci. 8: 113.

Brekhman,I.I.&I.V.Dardymov.1969.Pharmacological investigation of glycosides from ginseng and eleutherococcus. Lloydia 32: 46.

Brekhman, I.I., Ed. 1977. Adaptation and Adaptogens. Proceedings of the 2nd simposium: Processes of Adaptation and Biologically Active Substances (Vladivostok, May 1975). Far East Scientific Center of the USSR Academy of Sciences. Vladivostok. (Russian)

Brindley, D.N. & Y. Rolland. 1989. Possible connection between stress, diabetes, obesity, hypertension and altered lipoprotein metabolism that may result in atherosclerosis. Clin. Sci. 77: 453.

Brinkmann, A.O. 1994. Steroid hormone receptors: activators of gene transcription. J. Pediatr. Endocrinol. 7: 275.

Burman, B.G. & G. Margolin. 1992. Analysis of the association between marital relationships and health problems: An interactional perspective. Psychol. Bull. 112: 39.

Calogero, A.E. et al. 1996. Effects of corticotropin-releasing hormone on ovarian estrogen production in vitro. Endocrinology 137: 4161.

Chen, C.C. et al. 1995. Adverse life events and breast cancer: case-control study. Br. Med. J. 311: 1527.

Chiang, H.C., J.J. Wang & R.T. Wu. 1992. Immunomodulating effects of the hydrolysis products of formosanin C and beta-ecdysone from Paris formosana Hayata. Anticancer Res. 12: 1475.

Chrousos, G.P. & P.W. Gold. 1992. The concepts of

stress and stress system disorders: Overview of physical and behavioral homeostasis. JAMA 267: 1244.

Chrousos, G.P. 1997. The future of pediatric and adolescent endocrinology. Ann. N.Y. Acad. Sci. 816: 4.

Cicero, A.F. et al. 2004. Effects of Siberian ginseng (Eleutherococcus senticosus maxim.) on eldery quality of life: a randomized clinical trial. Arch. Gerontol. Geriatr. Suppl. 9: 69.

Ciolino, H.P., P.J. Daschner & G.C. Yeh. 1999. Dietary flavonols quercetin and kaempferol are ligands of the aryl hydrocarbon receptor that affect CYP1A1 transcription differentially. Biochem. J. 340: 715.

Cox, D.J. & L.A. Godner-Frederick. 1991. The role of stress in diabetes mellitus. In: Stress, Coping, and Disease. P.M. McCabe, N. Schneiderman, T.M. Field & J.S. Skyler, Eds. Earlbaum. Hillside, NJ. p. 118.

Das, D. & R.K. Banerjee. 1993. Effect of stress on the antioxidant enzymes and gastric ulceration. Mol. Cell. Biochem. 125: 115.

De Bock, K. et al. 2004. Acute Rhodiola rosea intake can improve endurance exercise performance. Int. J. Sport. Nitr. Exerc. Metab. 14:298.

Derventzi, A. & S.I.S. Rattan. 1992. Homeostatic imbalance during cellular aging: Altered responsiveness. Mutat. Res. 256: 191.

Drozd, J., Sawicka, T., Prosinska, J. 2002. Estimation of humoral activity of Eleutherococcus senticosus. Acta Pol. Pharm. 59: 395.

Eichenbaum, H. & T. Otto. 1992. The hippocampus - what does it do? Behav. Neurol. Biol. 57: 2.

Elizarov, E.N. & V.A. Khudoshin. 1977. Effect of physical exercises and Eleutherococcus on lipid metabolic indices in submariners. Voen. Med. Zh. 4: 64. (Russian)

Foster, S. 1999. No matter your physical state, adaptogens can help your body meet each day's challenges. Herbs for Health, May/June: 39.

Fulder S. 1980. The drug that builds Russians. New Scientist (21 August): 576.

Gagarinova, V.M. et al. 1990. The use of adaptogens of plant origin in protecting children against influenza and other acute respiratory diseases. Pediatriia 9: 108. (Russian)

Gerling, I. & O. Pribilla. 1986. Breath and blood alcohol concentration following intake of Eleutherococcus and Gallexier. Blutalkohol 23: 400. (in German)

Geyer, S. 1996. Social factor in the development and course of cancer. Cancer J. 9: 8.

Hagglof, B. et al. 1991. The Swedish childhood diabetes study: Indications of severe psychological stress as a risk factor for type I (insulin-dependent) diabetes mellitus in childhood. Diabetologia 34: 579.

Hajdu, Z. et al. 1998. A stilbene from the roots of leuzea carthamoides. J. Nat. Prod. 61: 1298.

Harris, R.A., M.S. Brodie & T.V. Dunwiddie. 1992. Possible substrates of ethanol reinforcement: GABA and dopamine. Ann. N.Y. Acad. Sci. 654: 61.

Heiser, I. & E.F. Elstner. 1998. The biochemistry of plant stress and disease: Oxygen activation as a basic principle. Ann. N.Y. Acad. Sci. 851: 224.

Hikino, H. et al. 1986. Isolation and hypoglycemic activity of eleutherans A, B, C, D, E, and G: glycans of Eleutherococcus senticosus roots. J. Nat. Prod. 49: 293.

House, J.S., K.R. Landis & D. Umberson. 1988. Social relationships and health. Science 241: 540.

Iaremenko, K.V. 1989. Adaptogens as means of the prevention of malignant tumors. Vopr. Onkol. 35: 912. (Russian)

Ikeya, Y. et al. 1979. The constituents of Schizandra chinensis Baill. I. Isolation and structure determination of five new lignans, gomisin A, B, C, F and G, and the absolute structure of schizandrin. Chem. Pharm. Bull. (Tokio) 27: 1383.

Ip, S.P., C.T. Che & K.M. Ko. 1998. Structure-activity relationship of schizandrins in enhancing liver mitochondrial glutathione status in CCl4-poisoned mice. Chung Kuo Yao Li Hsueh Pao 19: 313.

Jackson, T., A. Iezzi & K. Lafreniere. 1996. The differential effects of employment status on chronic pain and healthy comparison groups. Int. J. Behav. Med. 3: 354.

Ji, L.L. 1996. Exercise, oxidative stress, and antioxidants. Am. J. Sports Med. 24: 20.

Kamen, B. 1988. Siberian Ginseng. R.A. Passwater & E. Mindell, Eds. Keats Publishing, Inc.. New Canaan, CT.

Kaplan, J.R. et al. 1991. Role of sympathoadrenal medullary activation in the initiation and progression of atherosclerosis. Circulation 84 (Suppl. 6): VI 23.

Kerr, D.S. et al. 1991. Chronic stress-induced acceleration of electrophysiologic and morphometric biomarkers of hippocampal aging. J. Neurosci. 11: 1316.

Kelly, G.S. 2001. Rhodiola rosea: a possible plant adaptogen. Altern. Med. Rev. 6: 293.

Kiecolt-Glaser, J.K. et al. 1998. Marital stress: Immunologic, neuroendocrine, and autonomic correlates. Ann. N.Y. Acad. Sci. 840: 656.

Kimura, Y., Sumiyoshi, M. 2004. Effects of various Eleutherococcus senticosus cortex on swimming time, natural killer activity and corticosterone level in forced swimming stressed mice. J. Ethnopharmacol. 95: 447.

Kirschbaum, C. et al. 1995. Persistent high cortisol responses to repeated psychological stress in a subpopulation of healthy men. Psychosom. Med. 57: 468.

Kochetkov, N.K., A. Khorlin & O.S. Chizhov. 1961. Schizandrin - lignan of unusual structure. Tetrahedron Lett., 730.

Kochetkov, N.K. et al. 1962. Deoxyschizandrin - structure and total synthesis. Tetrahedron Lett., 361.

Kudriashov, Iu.B. & E.N. Goncharenko. 1999. Current problems of chemical radiation protection of organisms. Radiats. Biol. Radioecol. 39: 197. (Russian)

Kuiper, G.G. et al. 1998. Interaction of estrogenic chemicals and phytoestrogens with estrogen receptor beta. Endocrinology 139: 4252.

Lawler, K.A., Z.C. Wilcox & S.F. Anderson. 1995. Gender differences in patterns of dynamic cardiovascular regulation. Psychosom. Med. 57: 357.

Lebedev, A.A. 1971. Limonnik. Tashkent. (Russian)

Lee, I.S. et al. 1999. Structure-activity relationships of lignans from Schisandra chinensis as platelet activating factor antagonists. Biol. Pharm. Bull. 22: 265.

Lehman, C. et al. 1991. Impact of environmental stress on the expression of insulindependent diabetes mellitus. Behav. Neurosci. 105: 241.

Leibowitz, S.F. 1986. Bran monoamines and peptides: role in the control of eating behavior. Fed. Proc. 45: 1396.

Leshem, Y.Y. & P.J. Kuiper. 1996. Is there a GAS (general adaptation syndrome) response to various types of environmental stress? Biol. Plant 38: 1.

Lichtenthaler, H.K. 1996. Vegetation stress: An introduction to the stress concept in plants. J. Plant Physiol. 148: 4.

Lin, Y.J., L. Seroude & S. Benzer. 1998. Extended life-span and stress resistance in the Drosophila mutant methuselah. Science 282: 943.

Lindheim, S.R. et al. 1992. Behavioral stress responses in premenopausal and postmenopausal women and the effects of estrogen. Am. J. Obstet. Gynecol. 167: 1831.

Liu, J. & A. Mori. 1994. Involvement of reactive oxygen species in emotional stress: A hypothesis based on the immobilization stress-induced oxidative damage and antioxidant defense changes in rat bran, and the effect of antioxidant treatment with reduced glutathione. Int. J. Stress Manag. 1: 249.

Luger, A., et al. 1987. Acute hypothalamic-pituitary-adrenal responses to stress and treadmill exercises. Physiologic adaptation to physical training. N. Engl. J. Med. 316: 1309.

Lupandin, A.V. 1989. The role of catecholaminergic synapses in the mechanism of the formation of adaptation with the participation of polyphenol adaptogens. Fiziol. Zh. SSSR 75: 1082. (Russian)

Lupandin, A.V. 1990. The adaptation to extreme natural and technogenic factors in trained and untrained subjects under the influence of adaptogens. Fiziol. Cheloveka 16: 114.(Russian)

Maslova, L.V., Iu.B. Lishmanov & L.N. Maslov. 1993. Cardioprotective effects of adaptogens of plant origin. Bull. Eksp. Biol. Med. 115: 269. (Russian)

Malyszko, J. et al. 1994. Stress-dependent changes in fibrinolysis, serotonin and platelet aggregation in rats. Life Sci. 54: 1275.

Meerson, F.Z. 1983. The Failing Heart: Adaptation and Deadaptation. A.M. Katz, Ed. Raven Press, New York.

Meydani, M. & W.J. Evance. 1993. Free radicals, exercise, and aging. In: Free Radical in Aging. B.P. Y, Ed. CRC Press. Boca Raton, FL. p. 183.

Molokovskii, D.S., V.V. Davydov & V.V. Tiulenev. 1989. The action of adaptogenic plant preparations in experimental alloxan diabetes. Probl. Endocrinol. (Moscow) 35: 82. (Russian)

Mowrey, D.B. 1993. Siberian ginseng, eleuthero root. In: Herbal Tonic Therapies. Keats Publishing, Inc.. New Canaan, CT. p. 192.

Nomura, M. et al. 1994. Gomisin A, a lignan component of Schizandra fruits, inhibits development of preneoplastic lesions in rat liver by 3'-methyl-4-dimethylamino-azobenzene. Cancer Lett. 76: 11.

Opletal, L. et al. 1997. Phytotherapeutic aspects of diseases of the circulatory system. Leuzea carthamoides (WILLD.) DC: the status of research and possible use of the taxon. Ceska Slov. Farm. 46: 247.

Ovodov, Yu.S. et al. 1967. Glycosides of Eleutherococcus senticosus. II. Structure of eleutherosides A, B1, C and D. Khim. Prirodnih Soedin. 1: 63. (in Russian)

Peterson, W.C. 1994. Silent depression: the fate of the American dream. W.W. Norton & Company. New York. London.

Pollard, T.M., et al. 1995. Effect of academic examination stress on eating behavior and blood lipid levels. Int. J. Behav. Med. 2: 299.

Rabin, D. et al. 1998. Stress and reproduction: Physiologic and pathophysiologic interaction between the stress and reproductive axes. Adv. Exp. Med. Biol. 245: 377.

Razafimanalina, R., P. Mormede & L. Velley. 1996. Gustatory preference-aversion profiles for saccharin, quinine and alcohol in Roman high- and low-avoidance lines. Behav. Pharmacol. 7: 78.

Rebuffe-Scrive, M. et al. 1992. Effect of chronic stress and exogenous glucocorticoids on regional fat distribution and metabolism. Physiol. Behav. 52: 583.

Rogala, E. et al. 2003. The influence of Eleutherococcus senticosus on cellular and humoral immunological response of mice. Pol. J. Vet. Sci. 6 (suppl.): 37.

Rose, R.M., C.D. Jenkins & M. Hurst. 1982. Endocrine activity in air traffic controllers at work. I., II., III. Psychoneuroendocrinology 7: 101, 113, 125.

Roy, M.S. et al. 1993. The ovine corticotropin releasing hormone test in type I diabetic patients and controls: Suggestion of mild chronic hypercortisolism. Metabolism 42: 696.

Salikhova, R.A. et al. 1997. Effect of Rhodiola rosea on the yield of mutation alterations and DNA repair in bone marrow cells. Patol. Fiziol. Eksp. Ter. 4: 22. (in Russian)

Sapolsky, R., L. Krey & B.S. McEwen. 1986. The neuroendocrinology of stress and aging: The glucocorticoid cascade hypothesis. Endocrinol. Rev. 7: 284.

Saratikov, A.S. 1974. Golden Root. E.D. Goldberg, Ed. Tomsk University. Tomsk. (Russian)

Schleifer, S.J. et al. 1989. Depression and immunity: Role of age, sex, and severity. Arch. Gen. Psychiatry 46: 81.

Schwarzer, R. 1994. Optimism, vulnerability, and self-beliefs as health-related cognitions: A systematic overview. Psychol. Health 9: 161.

Sclafani, A. & A. Kirchgessner. 1986. The role of the median hypothalamus in the control of food intake: An update. In: Feeding Behavior, Neural and Humoral Controls. R.C. Ritter, S. Ritter & C.D. Barnes, Eds. Academic Press. New York. p. 27.

Selye, H. 1936. A syndrome produced by diverse nocous agent. Nature 138: 32.

Selye, H. 1946. The general adaptation syndrome and the diseases of adaptation. J. Clin. Endocrinol. 6: 117.

Shevtsov, V.A. et al. 2003. A randomized trial of two different doses of a SHR-5 Rhodiola rosea extract versus placebo and control of capacity for mental work. Phytomedicine. 10: 95.

So, F.V. et al. 1997. Inhibition of proliferation of estrogen receptor-positive MCF-7 human breast cancer cells by flavonoids in the presence and absence of excess estrogen. Cancer Lett 112: 127.

Sosnova, T.L. et al. 1984. Stimulating effects of eleutherococcus and Chinese schizandra used for prevention of visual fatigue during work connected with color discrimination. Gig. Sanit. 12: 7. (Russian)

Stunkard, A.J., T.T. Foch & Z. Hrubec. 1986. A twin study of human obesity. J. Am. Med. Assoc. 256: 51.

Surwit, R.S., S.L. Ross & M.N. Feinglos. 1991. Stress, behavior and glucose control in diabetes mellitus. In: Stress, Coping, and Disease. P.M. McCabe, N. Schneiderman, T. M. Field & J.S. Skyler, Eds. Earlbaum. Hillside, NJ. p. 97.

Szolomicki, J. et al. 2000. The influence of active components of Eleutherococcus senticosus on cellular defence and physical fitness in man. Phytother. Res. 14: 30.

Tarui, H. & A. Nakamura. 1991. Hormonal responses of pilots flying high- performance aircraft during seven repetitive flight missions. Aviat. Space Environ. Med. 62: 1127.

Tiukavkina, N.A., I.A. Rulenko & Iu.A. Kolesnic. 1996. Natural flavonoids as dietary antioxidants and biologically active additives. Vopr. Pitan. 2: 33. (Russian)

Toussaint, O. et al. 1998. Reciprocal relationship between the resistance to stresses and cellular aging. Ann. N.Y. Acad. Sci. 851: 450.

Tsigos, C. & P.G. Chrousos. 1995. Stress, endocrine manifestations and diseases. In: Handbook of Stress Medicine. C. L. Cooper, Ed., CRC Press. Boca Raton, FL. p. 61.

Udintsev, S.N., V.P. Schakhov & I.G. Borovsky. 1991. On the mechanism of differential effect of low dose adaptogens on the functional activity of normal and transformed cellular elements in vitro. Biofizika 36: 624. (Russian)

Vereshchagin, I.A., O.D. Geskina & E.R. Bukhteeva. 1982. Increased effectiveness of antibiotic therapy with adaptogens in dysentery and Proteus infection in children. Antibiotiki 27: 65. (Russian)

Vershinina, S.F. 1967. On the effect of Leuzea carthamoides extract and sarcolysin on the course of lympholeukosis in NK-Ly mice. Vopr. Oncol. 13: 99. (Russian)

Wildfeuer, A. & D. Mayerhofer. 1994. The effect of plant preparations on cellular functions in body defense. Arzneimittelforschung 44: 361. (German)

Yasukawa, K. et al. 1992. Gomisin A inhibits tumor promotion by 12-O-tetradecanoylphorbol-13-acetate in two-stage carcinogenesis in mouse skin. Oncology 49: 68.

Yung, L., E. Gordis & J. Holt. 1983. Dietary choices and likelihood of abstinence among alcoholic patients in and outpatient clinic. Drug Alcohol Depend. 12: 355.

Zhao, B.L. et al. 1990. Scavenging effect of schizandrins on active oxygen radicals. Cell. Biol. Int. Rep. 14: 99.

GLOSSARY

Adaptation syndrome – sum total of the changes raised in the body under stress.

Adaptogens – natural substances, which restore the nonspecific resistance of the body decreased by stressful conditions.

Adrenals – adrenal glands, which produce glucocorticoids in its cortex part and adrenaline and noradrenaline - in medulla part.

Aglicon – non-carbohydrate part of glycoside molecule.

Antioxidants – the substances capable to prevent damages of DNA, proteins and lipids by reactive oxygen species such as HO^*, O_2^-, H_2O_2 and others.

ATP – adenosinetriphosphate, the energy accumulator and energy carrier in all cells of the body.

Catecholaminergic neurotransmitters – dopamine, adrenaline and noradrenaline, which play the role of hormones and also transmitters of impulses in specific neurons and synapses.

Cellular immunity – immune response with participation of T lymphocytes.

Creatine phosphate – a high-energy phosphate-storage compound found in muscle.

Cytochromes – proteins, components of the electron transport system in mitochondria.

DNA – deoxyribonucleic acid – polymer in which genetic information is encoded.

Erythrocytosis – increased amount of erythrocytes.

Erythropenia – decreased amount of erythrocytes.

Estrogens – steroid female hormones.

Free radicals – an uncharged atoms or molecules that contain an unpaired electron and are highly reactive.

Glucocorticoids – steroid hormones (cortisol, cortison, corticosterone) produced by adrenal cortex; participate in adaptive response to stressors action.

Glutathione – a peptide, regulating the redox state of the cell.

Glycogen – the major storage form of carbohydrates mostly in muscles and liver.

Homeostasis – the state of dynamic equilibrium of all processes in the body that provides viability of the organism.

Hormone receptors – structure on cellular surface, which interact with certain hormone to initiate a characteristic response.

Hypoglycemia – low concentration of blood sugar.

Hyperglycemia – high concentration of blood sugar.

Hypotension – low blood pressure.

Hypoxia – shortage of oxygen.

Immune system – protective system of the organism, constituents of which are bone marrow, thymus gland, spleen, lymph nodes.

Leukocytosis – increased amount of leukocytes.

Leukopenia – decreased amount of leukocytes.

Metabolism – sum total of enzyme-catalyzed reactions, which provide viability of the cell. The products of particular reactions called metabolites. There are two opposite directions of metabolism: anabolism – synthesis of complex molecules and catabolism – degradation of complex molecules.

Mitochondria – cellular organelle, in which oxidative phosphorylation and ATP formation carried out; it is called also "energy plant".

Neuropeptide – short chain of amino acids produced and secreted by neural tissue.

Oxidative phosphorylation – the process of energy production and its accumulation in the form of ATP.

Oxygen radical – superoxide (O_2^-), highly reactive and toxic molecule formed mainly in mitochondria during oxidative reactions; with the help of special enzyme it converted to less harmful H_2O_2.

Pituitary gland – endocrine gland of brain connected with hypothalamus and produces number of peptide hormones, including adrenocorticotropin.

Prophylaxis – diseases prevention.

Steroids – lipids that contain four fused carbon rings and are derived from the molecule of cholesterol.

Synergic action – increase efficacy under joint action of some factors in comparison with their separate action.

Thyroid gland – endocrine gland produced thyroid hormone, which increases the basal metabolic rate of most cells in the body, has a protein anabolic effect and some others.

Vegetative nervous system – autonomic motor system, which regulates activity of some internal organs and some metabolic processes, providing homeostasis.

www.ingramcontent.com/pod-product-compliance
Lightning Source LLC
Chambersburg PA
CBHW020334290526
45785CB00005B/2016